Baby Steps

I'm diagnosed, now what?

Tyrus Hinton

Copyright © 2017 by Tyrus J. Hinton

All rights reserved. No part of this publication may be reproduced, distributed, or transmitted in any form or by any means, including photocopying, recording, or other electronic or mechanical methods, without the prior written permission of the publisher, except in the case of brief quotations embodied in critical reviews and certain other noncommercial uses permitted by copyright law.

Cover Design: Genesis Doubledee

Layout Design: Nicole DeSpain

Book Project Management: Start Write, Inc.

ISBN: 978-0-9987700-0-0

TABLE OF CONTENTS

Foreword	5
Introduction	9
Day 1: Just Breathe	11
Day 2: Listen, Listen, Listen!	17
Day 3: Find a Song	27
Day 4: Erase the Routine	33
Day 5: Just Journal It	41
Day 6: Blind Trust	49
Day 7: Let It All Out!	59
Day 8: Don't Cheat Yourself	65
Day 9: Treatment	75
Day 10: Neglect	81

FOREWORD

THERE ARE CERTAIN PEOPLE within our lifetime that we are fortunate and blessed enough come into contact – people that leave an indelible mark on us. Tyrus Hinton is one of those individuals for me. On the surface, Tyrus Hinton is an unassuming, laid back, courteous, and always gracious man of great faith. However, after closer examination, one quickly realizes that Tyrus is one of the most charismatic, dynamic, instinctive, relevant, thought-provoking, and influential change agents of this generation.

The way in which Tyrus is gifted to make authentic connections with virtually everyone that he comes into contact with is truly a divinely remarkable gift. It is within the scope of this gift that I am convinced that *Baby Steps* will have a lasting impact on people for generations to come. It is my personal belief that this book crosses cultural, racial, socioeconomic, generational, and religious divides.

Additionally, *Baby Steps* will compel everyone who reads it to reacquaint himself or herself with his or her own personal collection of memories about grief. While reading this book, I was reminded of an experience that my wife and I had during the birth of my son, Judah. My son was born three and a half months prematurely (26 weeks), and he and my wife were within minutes of death. Because of my limited life experience, I thought that grief was only reserved for death experiences because the only times that I had experienced grief was during the death of loved ones. However, I soon found out that grief was also heavily present in what I like to call "life suspended" situations as well.

I came within minutes of becoming a widower and a single parent. So for that period of my life, time felt as though it was literally suspended. I was sandwiched between devastating pain and divine providence.

Many reading this book will perhaps feel that same sense of time suspension. Nevertheless, I can say with great confidence that *Baby Steps* will be a heart-healing and mind-stabilizing tool for those dealing with the grief of an unfortunate diagnosis. I wish that my wife and I had had a book of this kind while going through our process. Nonetheless, I am grateful that such a comprehensive and systematic guide now exists.

I applaud Tyrus and his wife Tryphene for sharing their insight and experience with us. Not only do I strongly encourage the reading of this book, but I believe that this book should be shared throughout every hospital, clinic, and medical facility worldwide. Our journeys may be difficult, but we will arrive at brighter days.

Baby Steps

We all wish to make great strides, but this progression will start with *Baby Steps*. Read every word of this book. Then share it with the world!

Roger Green, Jr.
The Journey of Living Day by Day, Author

INTRODUCTION

There are so many things that happen in life to which we have no answers for. I believe that childhood illnesses are one of those things.

Baby Steps provides a practical day by day approach to a change in your entire family, routine and life which we had not planned for.

While there are many medical resources during our sons diagnosis and even early stages of treatment, we still had no clue what to expect or how to navigate through the toughest days that would lay ahead.

Medically everything was covered, but for the simple things like day to day emotional expectations, we had no direction. We eventually formed great relationships with other parents and staff which took time, but it would have been very helpful to have something in hand to kind of help us down the beginning path.

I don't promise that this will be the final outline for you, but can assure you that this resource will be helpful as you begin this journey with your child.

There will be a few chapters that you may have to refer to often. Do it and then help another family that will face the same challenge in days to come.

Cry, smile, scream, and do whatever you must, just remember that we have to get back in that room and be strong for the kids.

We have experienced everything written in this book and have big hopes that this will be a great resource for you in days to come.

Day 1

Just Breathe

Breathe...

You have just received one of the hardest hits that you could have ever possibly received. It is not your neighbor, it is not your best friend, it is not about someone else. This time, it is you. It is your family affected by devastation.

I know you don't need fancy words or kind gestures. They simply will not help. Trust me, I know. So don't even think about it. You don't have to put on a brave face. You don't have to worry about the bravado dad or mom; go ahead and let your makeup become a mess. This is a private moment. There are no crowds in the room. There are no lights, cameras and action. How you look is not important. Right now I know you are just trying to catch your breath and that is completely normal. You just took the hardest hit you never saw coming.

So pause, scream, or even cry if you need to, but when you are done, take another breath! Just inhale and exhale. Concentrate on trying to breathe again and again. Breathe in between the tears and disappointment.

I know you don't really even understand what is happening right now, but please, whatever you do, keep breathing. I read from a book of a popular speaker that upon dealing with an unbearable amount of tragedy, he took out a piece of paper and wrote a short letter to himself. It was only two words: "Just live."

Your breaths symbolize that you are choosing to live. You are choosing to reserve your strength for your child. I know it is easier said than done, and I am not even suggesting that you can take it all in at once, but take it from someone who has been where you are right now.

Take a walk. Get and up and walk up and down the hall. Go outside and breathe in some fresh air. I want you to know it is okay to take a moment for yourself. You just learned information that changed your life forever. Take some time to process it; you may have to completely tune everyone out or shut completely down. Your child needs your strength right now.

You will have time for being brave later, but for today. Just breathe.

Action Items:

The old adage is true: "Better to have it and not need it, rather than to need it and not have it."

I would like to suggest that you read two articles. One is a breathing exercise article by Dr. David Carbonell, also known as the "Anxiety Coach." The other article is on deep breathing and is written by David Rakal at psychecentral.com. I will include the links below. Understand that I am not trying to say that the stress that you are dealing with now is going to give you anxiety attacks or cause you to have a mental breakdown. What I am saying is that the trauma that you are experiencing and will experience in the coming days could cause your body to react similarly to how mine did, so I want to help you prepare.

That is what the following information and suggested activities are for you. I am listing the abdominal breathing exercise that is discussed in David Rakal's article. Due to space, I am only listing the exercise steps, but I do highly recommend you read both articles in their entirety. Dr. Carbonell actually does a demonstration on his site of the same exercise, which he refers to as "Belly Breathing." Please watch it if you are a visual learner, or have any trouble following the steps below:

- Place one hand on your chest and the other on your abdomen. When you take a deep breath in, the hand on the abdomen should rise higher than the one on the chest. This insures that the diaphragm is pulling air into the bases of the lungs.

- After exhaling through the mouth, take a slow deep breath in through your nose, imagining that you are sucking in all the air in the room, and hold it for a count of 7 (or as long as you are able, not exceeding 7).
- Slowly exhale through your mouth for a count of 8. As all the air is released with relaxation, gently contract your abdominal muscles to completely evacuate the remaining air from the lungs. It is important to remember that we deepen respirations not by inhaling more air, but through completely exhaling it.
- Repeat the cycle four more times for a total of 5 deep breaths, and try to breathe at a rate of one breath every 10 seconds (or 6 breaths per minute). At this rate, our heart rate variability increases which has a positive effect on cardiac health.

Remember, abdominal breathing is also known as diaphragmatic breathing. The diaphragm is a large muscle located between the chest and the abdomen.

Comfortable, deep breathing is the key to relaxation, so be sure to use this if you find it necessary!

Here are the article links for your reference and further research.

http://psychcentral.com/lib/learning-deep-breathing/

http://www.anxietycoach.com/breathingexercise.html

Also, please note, I'm no doctor, so if you have a medical, be sure to first consult with your physician before doing any techniques or anything that could interfere with your medical treatment. Your health is more important now than ever, so please be safe!

Day 2

Listen, Listen, Listen!

There is almost nothing more devastating than the sickness of your child. There are all sorts of traumas that we as humans are able to cope with, but serious illness of our children just isn't one of them. At first, it may seem like a nightmare that you cannot wake up from…next it is a reoccurring nightmare that you cannot escape. Once your brain accepts the facts that this crisis is real and is really happening to you, then you are ready to face it.

Don't suppress the pain. It will only hurt you in the end. You have to face the pain and begin to channel it in the best way possible…listening to everyone connected to the situation is critical. Listening enables you to make informed decisions and stay focused on the most important person in this situation—your beloved child who is suffering right now.

Again, I am talking to you from experience. I still remember our "diagnosis" day. It is actually a day I will never forget. Before "diagnosis" day, my wife and I both remember the countless fevers and multiple trips to the ER. At the time we believed that our young son must have had an ear infection, and/or possibly even a cold that wouldn't just get better. There many times that we dropped him off to daycare with a prescription and Tylenol for days at a time. We always believed it would come to an end soon. It actually got worse. There were short naps that ended with uncontrollable, violent screaming which scared the life out of all of us. We recall trying to soothe him by rocking him to get him to calm down. We would sing to him until he would settle down some, and then eventually we would return to what became "normal" for us.

Upon the approaching "diagnosis" day, we went into the doctor's office armed with the feedback from all of our son's caregivers. The information that we had obtained from both the daycare teachers and grandparents was crucial. That is the reason it is important that you listen to everything and everyone that is directly connected to this situation. Even the information from the other toddlers was helpful. All of this information that we were able to relay to the physicians was essential in learning the true cause of our son's symptoms.

When you have gathered all the information and there is an indication that a serious condition is forming or has formed, it is imperative that you prepare for the information that the doctors are getting ready to share with you and your family. Here are few things to do to prepare for diagnosis day:

First, Lean In – come close.

It has been said that the worst hit is the one that you never see coming. The punch will make you feel as if you just want to throw up! I totally get it and I have been there too. You cannot let that feeling allow you to zone out.

Next, take a minute if you need to take one. Ask the doctor to pause for a minute. A good way to prolong the minute is to ask to retrieve an IPad, notebook or start a Note in your phone.

Just know—it is important that you listen and take notes when the doctors are speaking to you.

Be sure to write down the information that you are hearing. It is impossible to digest it all at one time. You will not be able to get all the information word by word, so just be sure to write down key words and terms, things that you have never heard before so that you can research them in between the tears.

Lastly, tune in and listen to the treatment plan that they are presenting to you. It will be necessary to remember the side effects and details to share with your family and support system. The side effects can be scary, but it will be much easier to prepare for them if your support group is aware of the details as well.

In order to prepare for the journey ahead, "listening" will be a skill in which you must become super-efficient. Here is a list of things that will help you listen:

1. Do your best to put your emotions aside.

   This is a critical time in your life and the life of your child. It will be impossible for you to not display emotions at all, but for now it will key for you to check your emotions long enough gain the critical information from all parties involved to make informed decisions for the journey ahead.

2. Try to listen more than you talk.

   There will be plenty of time for you to share your feelings and emotions with others, but right now is not that time. You need to focus on information-gathering more than information- sharing. Try not to interrupt. It will be important for the speaker to get out his or her thoughts to you without being interrupted. Keep in mind that although it is your child, it is not easy for the person sharing to give you the information.

3. Prepare yourself to listen.

    We are taught in so many other areas of life that "preparation is a key of success," however we often do not apply this rule with listening. Take a few minutes and clear your mind. Relax and get ready to take in the information that is being given to you. Grab a notebook or journal to be able to make notes while the speaker is sharing. This will also aid in your ability to refer back to the conversation later or ask follow-up questions. This may be a good time to practice any type of mediation with which you are familiar.

4. Be attentive, focus and remove all distractions.

    In an age of endless technology and 24/7 media, it is critical to remove distractions while you are listening to critical content.

The information that is being shared with you is already difficult to hear and process, so the last thing you need is anything that makes it easier for you to lose focus and/or zone out.

Action Items:

List the ways that you are already a good listener:

_____

_____

_____

_____

_____

_____

_____

List your "listening" challenges:

_____

_____

_____

_____

_____

_____

_____

What item will be the best way for you to record and keep track of information on the journey:

_____ Electronic Device

_____ Notebook/Journal

If you did not choose electronic device, make an appointment for yourself below to get the notebook/journal:

DAY:_____

DATE:_____

TIME:_____

STORE:_____

Who will be your accountability partner on this journey to make sure that you are helping yourself by putting these tools into practice:

NAME: _____

Give yourself an appointment to reach out to this person:

DAY:_____

DATE:_____

TIME:_____

METHOD:

_____ EMAIL

_____ TEXT

_____ CALL

_____ SOCIAL MEDIA MESSENGING CHANNEL

Day 3

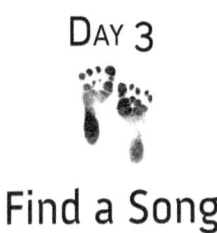

Find a Song

One of the most powerful tools of coping that we can ever experience is music. Music can suspend you in time, take you to another place, transform your mind, and touch your soul.

One of the best ways to stake claim on your sanity is to introduce music to your journey as quickly as you can. "Diagnosis" day hit us pretty hard.

After the doctors explained the treatment plan, the journey began almost immediately.

Our son was bombarded with pain medications, which left him crying uncontrollably and completely miserable. We wanted to console him, and we did our best, but it was the most challenging thing we had ever faced. The doctors had left us in the room to digest the news. We were sitting there, our world completely rocked and us literally speechless. We learned that day that our baby boy had AML—acute myeloid leukemia.

The term "acute" refers to the tendency of this disease to progress rapidly. The second term in its name — myelogenous — which distinguishes it from a disorder of the lymphocytes. This disease attacks the body rapidly, and unlike other cancers, AML does not occur in stages. Instead, it tends to be found spread throughout the bloodstream at the time of diagnosis, and may have invaded an organ. As a result of its ability to affect the whole body at once, it must be treated aggressively as soon as possible.

You can imagine this news hit us like a ton of bricks. My wife stepped into the bathroom to silently scream, if that's even possible. I took my son, sat with him in the rocking chair and looked out the window. As I began to rock him, something amazing happened. We began singing "I Believe I Can Fly." My son's part in the song was singing the word "fly." I was holding on to the part that said "because I believe in miracles." We sang it over and over until we felt an indescribable type of peace. This moment would become a routine part of journey in the days to come.

Who knew that we would need that song on a daily basis? It has been said that music has the ability to touch us. Some people merely only hear music, others actually feel it. We are the latter. We allowed the song to alleviate our pain and usher us to a place of peace.

Often, when times would get tough and more challenging news would come to us, we would just start singing our song. When he was in excruciating pain, and his little body got weak, he still managed to gain enough strength to sing our song. On days when I just could not wrap my mind around why this was happening to me, to my son, to my family, I learned to just sing my song. Our song became our place of peace and solace on the most challenging days.

In addition to selecting a song for you and your family, you should consider assembling musical selections to play during treatments and difficult times. An online article from the American Psychological Association states:

"There is growing scientific evidence showing that the brain responds to music in very specific ways," says Lisa Hartling, PhD, professor of pediatrics at the University of Alberta and lead author of the study. "Playing music for kids during painful medical procedures is a simple intervention that can make a big difference." It worked wonders for us.

Music can be helpful for your entire family during this challenging time. Prevention magazine reports that clinical studies and anecdotal evidence from music therapists suggest that the sound of music:

- Can manage pain
- Can reduce the need for sedatives and pain relievers during and after surgery
- Can decreases nausea during chemotherapy
- Can relieve anxiety
- Can ease depression

These are all reasons to make music a part of the challenging journey that you and your family are currently facing.

Action Items:

What is a song that you can sing with your child that both of you can sing together?

_____

Is there a certain part that is easier for the child to remember, such as the chorus or special part? If yes, list here. If no, assign your child one or two words in the song to become "his or her part."

_____
_____
_____
_____

What are some songs that bring you peace that you can meditate on during difficult times?

_____

_____

_____

_____

_____

_____

Give yourself an appointment to put those songs in a playlist that is quickly accessible to you. (It can be on an Ipod, your phone, a CD, or anything else that works for you.)

Day: _____

Date:_____

Time: _____

Device Type: _____

Accountability Partner to make sure that I keep this appointment

_____

(Name)

Day 4

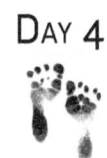

Erase the Routine—Life Change

REMEMBER THAT PUNCH TO the gut for which I told you to prepare? Well, that is the first of many. The stomach punch just changed your entire life. We realized that our schedules would never be the same, but we just didn't have any idea just how intense and drastic the change would be! During the time we learned of our son's condition, we had two other children. Our three small children were all eleven months apart, and they all still required care. The only constant that remained in our schedule was daycare drop-off and pick-up of our other two children. Other than that, our world was turned completely upside down. Dinner times were now sporadic and often had at least two people missing from the table due to hospitalization. One of us would go care for our son and the other had to stay to care for the other two children. Our social lives became non-existent. We could no longer hang out with families with other small children as our son's immune system just could not handle it. This also excluded family functions. We had to keep our family contained for the most part just to keep our son's exposure to germs and other factors as low as absolute possible.

Work continued because we still had financial obligations that had to be met, but scheduling was seriously adjusted to meet the "around-the-clock" needs of our baby boy. All extra spending ceased immediately. All scarce "leftover money" became our hospital/gas fund. All of this change occurred rapidly. We had to embrace the change quickly and keep on moving.

The changes not only affected us, but our two small children as well. They became medical assistants with us. We included them in the information process, showing them pictures in pamphlets and booklets (we did not have the Internet and all the technology available today) and taught them how to be cautious of everything that could have an adverse effect on their baby brother.

Keys to Embracing the "Erased Routine/ Changed Lives"

1. Involve the entire family! Let everyone know what is going on (ages of the other siblings will dictate how much information you give them and when you share it, but everyone needs to be made aware on some level).
2. If you have older children, create some times for them to spend with friends and enjoy some of their recreational activities. Enlist the support of family and friends to help you achieve this. You do not want these older

children/teens to grow resentful of the child that is battling a chronic condition. Peer relationships are important and can help them cope with the situation better. Coping skills are important for the entire family.

3. Coping 101- The difference between families/couples who survive life with a child battling a chronic or life-threatening illness and the ones who don't comes down to this one word: COPING. You all must develop healthy methods to deal with the ongoing difficult. On Day 2 we shared about finding a song and creating a playlist. You must have coping methods as an individual; you and your spouse will need coping strategies as a couple; and you will all need them as a family. They are imperative to structure of you all remaining intact and not unraveling under the pressure and stress.

4. Carve out 10-20 minutes a day to talk to your other children. Children also may resent the sick child if they feel as though they

no longer matter. You must not neglect these children during this time of crisis.

5. Don't forget self-care. You will not good to anyone else if you let yourself get completely rundown. It is like the emergency speech from the flight attendants: "In case of a real life threatening situation, place your mask on before trying to assist others." You will have to make yourself a priority in some ways. It actually is not an option. You have to remain healthy mentally, emotionally and physically.

6. Assemble a support network, you will need it. You need people that you can delegate tasks to that others can do. In some instances, you will be the only one who can help your sick child but if one of your other children is going to stay involved in a sport or extra-curricular activity a neighbor or friend may provide rides for your child for a season until you are able to resume those duties.

What is the most difficult adjustment for you with the schedule changes?

_____

Who can help you make this transition better?

_____

What are some ways that you can assist your children with the schedule change?

_____

What are some ways you can still spend time together as a couple during this difficult time?

_____

_____

_____

Make a list of people you can depend to become a part of your Support Team during this time? (There can be more than one group)

_____

_____

_____

_____

_____

_____

Who will be your accountability partner(s) to make sure you stay healthy and are taking care of you during this time?

Accountability Partner #1

_____

Accountability Partner #2

_____

Day 5

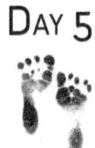

Just Journal It: Write It All Down

Napkins, receipts, discharge papers, backs of medication print-outs were our friend. That was the only way we could keep up with the constant changing information. Write down your questions. Don't try to organize, just write. As you continue to wrap your mind around all of the changes that are occurring in your life and the lives of your affected family members, there is something else that I found helpful that I would like to share with you.

It is important that you keep record of your days throughout this process. One of the best ways to do this is to journal. Journaling is not only helpful to help you keep track of notes and information, it also has proven to be very therapeutic.

As an information tracker, your journal can help you keep all the information that is rapidly coming at you in one place. Trust me, without one, you may find yourself like us writing on napkins, little scraps of paper, and on the back of discharge papers.

You are already experiencing high level of stress, and the last thing you need is to be walking around trying to find a little piece of paper that you wrote information on that you need. So do yourself a favor and get a couple of composition notebooks. Keep one in your car and one at home. That way you know that the vital information that you are keeping track of is in either one of the two places. Also, use those smart phones!

The second reason that journaling is helpful is because as you write things down it will help you retain important information for later. Some parents have children who are blessed with a full recovery. Journaling your experience helps you count your blessings, and can also be helpful if you find yourself encouraging another family later who is going through what you and your family survived.

For families whose loved one's illness whose goes into remission and returns, the journal is helpful as a reference as what worked before and what did not. Tracking side effects of certain medications, or how long it took for a particular treatment to take effect can be good information to have at another time.

Lastly, it is good to journal to track your own feelings and emotions. Some days it will be two words, such as, "This sucks," or, "Better today." Some people write angry letters, while others write their prayers, hopes and expectations. You cannot mess it up. It is yours. Whatever helps you get through the process is the most important thing. It is a place where you can write in vivid detail the events and how they made you feel. Sometimes you find yourself being the strong one so you don't share. This is a place where you can share all of your pent up frustrations, your inner rage, as well as your prayers for a miracle. You can write how one day was amazing and your baby slept through the night, or how horrible another night was because he or she awoke every hour on the hour screaming in pain.

It is also a place where you can list your expectations and hopes. You can use start with sentences like…

Today was a rough day because _____

_____

Last night was great because _____

_____

I am hoping for _____

_____

These are just a few sentence prompts to get you started. You will be surprised how easy the rest will flow after a while.

Action Items

1. Go get yourself a couple of journals. Give yourself a deadline to have it by _____.
2. If you absolutely hate writing on paper, consider these other journaling formats:
   - Keep notes in your phone or tablet by typing them.
   - Keep notes on your computer (if you are someone who always has it with you).
   - Keep audio notes (if you prefer to talk out your feelings and notes).
   - Start a blog. If you want to help others and you are not as concerned with privacy, you can always share your experience in blog/online format (you can still control who has access to it, in some instances, but this definitely is the least private method).

Baby Steps

3. Be consistent about when you journal. Try to set a specific time to journal, when specifically writing about your feelings and emotions. If you are information tracking, then you of course would do that as needed. Write a time and day that you will definitely journal: _____

4. Set a time limit (if necessary) _____ This will help it seem more like an appointment you set with yourself.

5. Make sure you log the time and date of each entry. It will be useful for you later to look back and see the time and date that specific events took place.

6. Remember those writing prompts from above? Be sure to use them if you need help getting inspired for your writing on that particular day:

    Today was a rough day because _____.
    Last night was great because _____.
    I am hoping for _____.

7. Think of journaling like a friend and openly share. The more comfortable you are, the more it will help you.
8. Read back from your journal often. It will help you see your journey and gain an appreciation of the good times, and encourage you to keep pushing on.

Day 6

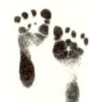

Blind Trust
(Build your support team)

Unless others in your family have dealt with childhood cancer, they will not understand the ups and downs of this debilitating disease. As well-meaning as your family may try to be, they generally will not by equipped to handle the totality of what your immediate family is really going through. Unfortunately, they don't understand that this is not like a cold which will go away in a few days. The question asked so often is, "So, when are you guys going home?" This question further proves the lack of understanding that many of our closest family members have about cancer. Often, we were asked questions that we didn't have the answers to, and this inability further frustrated us. Therefore, it became very necessary for us to reach out beyond our familiar circle of family and friends.

One of the ironies of the situation that you are facing is that you would think such a challenge would be a time in which you bond with family members beyond your immediate circle. In some instances that is true, but in reality, this is the time when you have to let down your guard and trust strangers, who often show more compassion and support.

Even if you have family in the medical profession, but they are not trained in the exact illness as your child, then you still have to feed them out of a "long-handled spoon," as the older folks used to say.

Also realize that some will not have the strength to handle day-day-day difficulties that your family is dealing with. Unfortunately, some people do not endure their own challenging times that well, especially when they don't understand. So I admonish you to do yourself and them a favor by not confiding and relying on them.

Actually, the exact opposite happened. We learned to trust complete strangers and look to them for hope and understanding. First, we had to trust the team of oncologists. We knew nothing; consequently we spent a lot of time learning about our son's condition and waiting in hospitals. Sometimes, we would sit there with our son; other times, we would explore the hospital. It was on our walks down the halls that we began to say, "Hello" to other families. Conversations about treatment plans, shared meals, pains, plans, victories, defeats, the good, bad and ugly, took place daily. Hallway conversations with other families became our norm. We were the only ones that could understand code leukemia. We almost became little doctors and nurses. We shared what we had because we realized that most days, we were all the hope that we had. This was before the **Health Insurance Portability and Accountability** Act of 1996 (**HIPAA**), Public **Law** went into effect. In addition, we knew each other's children and what was going on with them in case we had to help out one another.

We didn't know what else to do. Keep in mind that we were not living in the digital metropolis in which we are living now. There were no iPads, tablets, or cell phones to hold our attention. After reading and watching Barney, Elmo, and Sesame Street, we needed to step out of the room. What we did not have externally, my wife and I had to get from one another. Let me stop right here and say that if you and your significant other are already having a rough time, this kind of crisis has the potential to destroy your relationship.

While you are putting your child's care into the hands of doctors, you must take some time to make sure that your hearts are safe in one another's hands. If your relationship is struggling, you may have to find some time for counseling. This decision could have been much harder back when our son was sick, but I want to encourage you to do what we did: open up, talk to people, adjust your face, fix your tone, and you will be surprised how many folks are waiting to share info and even assist you in what is a hard time for them also. We did it, and even now, we are still reaching back to families to provide emotional support. I also encourage you to explore all the options available (Google Chat, Skype, etc.) to do whatever you have to do to hold onto your love. We didn't have these options available to us during our time. Your child needs you both now more than ever.

So many times, my wife and I needed independent emotional support. While we were there for one another all the time, there were days, while together, we were on a downward spiral because of the series of discoveries that the doctors had found. It always seemed as if we had conquered one obstacle, only to discover another one. This process demanded energy outside of us to get us through this painful ordeal. You will need the same. You cannot do this alone.

If you are a single parent and are facing this crisis without the support of the other biological parent, that is a tough situation to be in, for you are not going to be able to do this alone. The load is much too heavy for an individual to carry alone. It almost broke our backs, and there were two of us! So make sure that you are not facing this ordeal all by yourself. Married couples have each other to share their experience with each other and to help each other through difficult times. Since you don't have that built in, it is going to be even more crucial to you to get to know the other families who are facing the same struggle. Those are people that you can share your experiences with, both good and bad. Keep in mind that every day will not be bad; just condition yourself so that when the bad days come, you are ready.

We established relationships with the other families, which helped us with balance on this emotional roller coaster ride. We found it to be a good thing to have some people to share a laugh on good days, and a good cry when things were challenging.

It would be a huge benefit to you if you are able to do what we did.

We got to know each other, exchanged numbers, and looked for one another during our hospital stays. We stay in touch with one another now, and it has been over seventeen years since diagnosis day for us. Nurses, CNA's, and housekeepers even remain a part of our family. We knew what they liked; they knew when they were needed. They were so kind, compassionate, and gave us truly what we needed the most—an ear. There are some days on which you will just need to talk. Never underestimate the value of a great medical team. It seemed as though after they realized the type of news we would receive, they figured out not only the gentlest way to in-form us, but then they all followed that up by providing amazing support. Just know that there are some staff members who become so close to your family that the trauma may temporarily even affect them to the point of understanding when they have to step out of the room. Even they know when to take a break from troubling developments. They taught us a valuable lesson: sometimes, you just have to take a break from it.

You must learn to develop a support team with the people around you who are equipped to help you understand and assist you in managing all aspects of life during your family's challenging time.

Action Items:

1. Make sure you spend time with your significant other, and work on "being there" for one another. Get counseling if you need to, but if you guys are having problems, even more focus should be placed on the child, who needs you the most.

2. If you are a single parent, be sure to gather a few people that you trust and can truly depend on to support you during this time. Except in cases of abuse or neglect, you should reach out to the biological parent and give him/her an opportunity to be a part of the process, if your situation allows. Some illnesses are genetic or are linked to certain DNA factors. In such cases, it could be helpful to your child's condition to have access to the persons with both gene pools.

3. Be friendly. Everyone on your ward, on your floor, in the wing of your hospital, has a child going through some sort of devastating crisis. Some are more severe than others, but everyone is going through his/her own hardship. Smiling, speaking, or just making eye contact, are ways to show people that you are open to conversation or support. You won't "vibe" with everyone, but some of the people who ended up being closest to us, we came to know by one of these simple gestures.

4. Be understanding toward the staff. Unless you perceive your child to be in danger or someone is guilty of a mal-practice level offense, just remember that many hospitals are understaffed. We ended up receiving amazing, above-and-beyond service for our son just as a result of being understanding.
5. Get to know the dynamics of the hospital staff makeup. Learn who the hardest working staff members are; learn who is lazy. Ask questions of the staff as you befriend them. Someone will always give you the "lay of the land." That is important because you don't want to build your team with the wrong people. You need staff that is dedicated, compassionate, honest, and with a good bedside manner on this team you are secretly assembling. This "inside" info can be critical later. You can adjust procedures and treatments around your "preferred" medical staff's schedule. Even though you want to be nice, you still have an obligation to seek the highest level of care for your son or daughter.

DAY 7

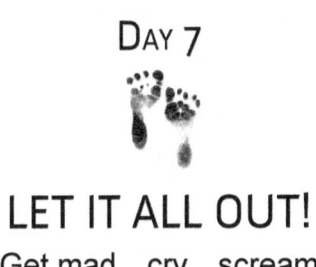

LET IT ALL OUT!
(Get mad…cry…scream)

No matter how many days pass, you will inevitably find yourself back at the "Why Me?" point. You will find yourself again asking the same nagging questions:

"Why me?"

"Why my kid?"

"Why my family?"

"What did I do wrong?"

Then, the inner rage kicks in:

"We didn't hurt anyone!"

We don't deserve this."

All of a sudden, every emotion imaginable hits you like a ton of bricks. It hit us so hard that some days we felt as if we could barely move. The reality takes a toll on you, and you move a little slower. We zoned out a lot when people were talking to us. Many days, I got in my car and arrived at my destination and didn't have any recollection of the drive. I wasn't even sure how I made it. Well, when you get to this point, you have to do what is natural for anyone in your shoes: get mad, scream, yell, cry, and repeat it until you feel better. The key is not to yell at people, or become "unglued" in front of your child. Your child will think that you blame him/her for his/her sickness, or worse, that you have given up hope. Remember, they are experiencing the same thing, but on a kid level. They don't know why this is happening to them either. So whatever you do must be strong for them. But in your alone time, in your private moments you must take off that superman cape you figuratively must wear all the time for your family, significant other and your baby. That is not the requirement. You must be human. Emotions are a clear symbol of humanity.

You cannot however, allow your emotions to rule you. There are too many people depending on you for that.

So you must find coping mechanisms for processing your emotions. I suggest that you meditate which is a mental exercise and combine this with some physical activity that allows for release.

Let's start with clearing your mind and meditation. Meditation just means to get quiet and posture yourself in an environment that is calming and allows for you to mentally collect your thoughts and emotions. Meditation allows you to bring your inner man, mind and body back in harmony with one another. It may sound weird, but our body is an amazing machine. It has many facets that allow for self-healing. We just have to know how to jump start those features. Meditation is one of those ways that we can control our emotions until we can get to a completely private place and let it all out as we described above. If you are spiritual or religious, meditation for you may be similar to praying to a higher power. Whatever works best for you is what we are suggesting you do.

The next step is physical release. We mentioned earlier that sometimes we walked up and down the halls. There would be other parents who came in their sweats and would take a jog or run around the hospital while the other parent was on duty. Some people learn boxing. Hitting a boxing bag is a great stress reliever. If that is too intense for you, you may try yoga or a fitness class. Engaging in physical activity is a great way to channel the emotion and stress during an ongoing challenging situation. So please, do yourself a favor a get a routine that works for you! If nothing else, sometimes you may have to go into the bathroom and scream into a pillow to muffle the sound! Whatever you do don't keep it bottled up. That is no good for anyone.

Action Items:

1. Don't be a superhero! When is the last time you truly let out your emotions?

   _____

   _____

2. Have you given yourself an opportunity to release all the anger and pain inside? If not, why? Who can you reach out to so that you can be accountable for taking the time to release? List them here and give yourself a deadline to reach out to them. Make an appointment with yourself

Person: _____

Date: _____

Time: _____

Person: _____

Date: _____

Time: _____

3. If you have let your emotions out, how will you best continue to manage your emotions? (Select as many as you think will work for you)

   ___Meditation—Quietly Listening to Music

   ___Meditation—Quiet Time During a Massage

   ___Meditation—Prayer to a Higher Power

   ___Meditation—Quiet Time during Journaling

   ___Physical Activity: Boxing Bag

   ___Physical Activity: Fitness Class

   ___Physical Activity: Running/Jogging

Day 8

Don't Cheat Yourself

It amazes me how much things have changed, even in my relatively short life. There have been so many technological advancements and medical breakthroughs since we battled with AML. I can remember when the expression "You've Got Mail" became popular in the 90's. The Internet was just becoming personalized and "user friendly." It was not nearly as advanced as it is now. The ability to connect over Wi-Fi was not available. I am talking about dialup modems.

This was a time where if your phone rang, you could get kicked off the Internet! Some of you may or may not remember the dial-up era. It was called "dial-up" because you could literally hear the modem dialing to connect you to the internet. AOL was at its prime during this time.

I am only forty-one now, but the information in the above paragraph just shows you how far technology has come since my early twenties. The closest thing I had to a smart phone was my beeper, while some folks had car phones, which could be detached and carried in a special bag. Now we have smart phones, but at the time I did not have a clue that the technology readily available would ever exist! For some, it is fascinating to have Internet access on our phones and tablets. The way we did our research and gathered additional information was through pamphlets distributed by the hospital, lending libraries, and the public library. I would read for hours, learn about another aspect of treatment and then have to another research an additional resource to gain a complete understanding. There never seemed to be any quick and readily available information. We also learned a great deal by asking questions of whatever families who would share information that they may have gained during the process also.

I remember having the option to believe the information presented to me by the doctor, or to travel to another doctor and ask for a second opinion. This practice was usually the culture of the 90's when my son was diagnosed. Thinking back about different opinions, I one hundred percent support getting additional information and/or a second opinion. Remember that this is your baby you are considering. I have discovered that most reputable doctors recommend it. If your city is smaller and its doctors are not dealing with a volume of childhood cancer cases, you may need to travel outside your city/town. At that time, we lived in New York and had access to some of the best oncologists. We had even considered and had applied to being a part of a clinical trial in California, however, our family was not accepted. As we began to connect with other parents, we learned about support groups. The support groups also were able to validate to us that we had the best possible physicians treating our child. I strongly suggest that you find someone or some group to connect with in your hospital or treatment center; they will be some of your best resources. I am not suggesting that they will have any more information than the professionals, but I do know that they can provide the emotional support you need. We were very fortunate. Our son's medical team was amazing and had extensive education. We reached out in every direction to get the best results. Search out the best. Remember that is your baby!

Today, you don't have to worry with the lack of information and resources that caused us to have to live with the limited information we were given. Even with the best health insurance, no one in our family, tracing back several generations, had encountered anything like this. In many cases, we just had to settle and make peace with the information as it was given to us. That is not your situation. Make sure that you read the information you are given by the medical team, and that you are following what you believe to be the expertise of the physicians. However, these days, you have far more access at your fingertips and for more information and resources.

Don't cheat yourself out of learning about the disease and drugs used to treat the illness. Make yourself familiar with the medical terminologies and alternative treatment plans. Be certain that you understand all of the side effects and complications that could arise before you decide if you want to participate in the clinical trial of a treatment plan, or if you want to go with the traditional treatment plans. Remain aware that every child responds differently to each treatment. Your child may be like our son and skip many of the anticipated side effects. If you are too tired to make a decision, clear your head before giving an answer. It is always a life-or-death situation with your baby. Therefore, take a minute, and be sure that your family is not making a hasty decision because of the overwhelming stress and emotions. Always make informed decisions that you have taken the time to research thoroughly. There is simply too much information available to you for you not to be well informed. Remember to use your journals and handheld devices to track the information presented so that you can research it.

Again, we cannot stress it enough: look for support groups. In most areas they are readily accessible and with technology the groups are much easier to find now. I remember another family sharing some information with us that prompted us to mention it to the doctor. It a great move for us. These days, you have much more access to information than we did. You may be able to search via Internet and find out so many facts. You can even search for what city can offer you the best care. We were in New York, as I mentioned earlier, but we have met people from small towns in North Carolina who drive two, three or four hours to get treated at UNC Chapel Hill hospitals because the area where they lived could not treat their cancer victim. You have an obligation to your child and your family to research. Do your own homework on the diagnosis, and get a second opinion (if you can).

Action Items:

1. **Take some time, and research your child's diagnosis.** Make two columns in your notebook. One column should be labeled "PERSONAL RESEARCH," and the other should be labeled "FOR FOLLOW-UP." The personal research may be things that will be helpful to you and your family for your particular case. The follow-up category should be a list from which you ask the doctor or medical team more questions that will help you understand better.

2. **Research the best cities for treating your child's illness.** Make sure that you write this information down, and write down contact numbers of these facilities just in case you need to reach out or transfer your child. These also could be places from which you could receive a second opinion.
3. **Take some time to research the treatments and medications available to your child.** Again, you can create those same two categories: one should be labeled "PERSONAL RESEARCH," and the other "FOLLOW-UP." The personal research may consist of things that will be helpful to you and your family for your particular case. The follow-up category should comprise of a list that you ask the doctor or medical team more questions to help you understand better.
4. **Research, ask, and look for support groups.** Write down contact names of group leaders and meeting locations. Find one that is a good fit for you. Make notes about what you

like and don't like about them. This listing may help you suggest one of the groups you learn about to someone else. Just because it is not a fit for you doesn't mean it won't be a good fit for someone else.

Day 9

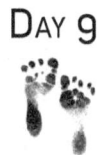

Treatment (It Helps and Hurts)

So everything we have been discussing in the last couple of days has been relatively mild. Now, get ready, because this next topic is not an easy one. *Treatment* can feel like a huge kick in the stomach.

Treatment is easy to understand, yet the side effects can be challenging to digest. The taste of medicine, to me, was horrible when I was growing up. So much has changed over the course of time, however. Children now like taking medicine because it tastes like candy and bubble gum. Years ago, we knew medicine was good for us is because it tasted so bad. For example, we used to be given castor oil! Even as children, we knew that there could be no other possible reason to digest something that was so horrendous unless it could make us feel better.

Well, that is how treatment is. The thing that would help our son get better would make him so sick throughout the entire process. Talk about unavoidable. You really hope for the best, but you almost have to prepare for the worst. We hoped for three days of chemo and assumed that we would be able to head home after. We planned for one-day stays. We only planned for the Hickman Broviack (Mediport) to remain in place and not have to be moved. All of the things that seemed so cut-and-dry were never that way. The length of time was challenging to pin down. There came a point that we decided to pack extra items and be prepared to stay. All of our plans were centered on treatment and the possibility of fever. The effects of the treatment were also unknown to us initially. We were not prepared for what happened next, however.

Our son's skin color changed with radiation treatment. He suffered hair loss because of medication (except for one patch, which we claimed represented his fight). Treatment can be very hash at times. Some days, our son was so weak that we had to carry him. He had no strength to walk. Some days, he walked into radiation, some days we carried him. Some days he would go in the machine alone, some days we had to hold him. Many days, we had to stand outside the room (because of radiation levels) and hear him screaming for us. This was not what we anticipated for our son. Again, we were very fortunate to have the staff take such a liking to our family.

We are not telling you this to frighten you. We just want you to be aware that it helps and hurts. We don't want you to be caught off guard by the possibilities. My hope for you is that your baby is so tough that he or she bypasses the majority of the side effects. If you have a good medical team, it will do a decent job of preparing you, but if you have a staff that is shy about details, then you could really have some difficult moments for which you are not prepared. Again, that is why it is important to research and be actively engaged in your child's treatment, not to be an obstruction, but so you are prepared, and that your child doesn't undergo anything that is not absolutely necessary.

Action Items

1. Meditate. Be sure to take quiet time alone before and after the treatments when possible. I once was told that sometimes to administer self-care, you have to become a minute-thief. Sometimes, you cannot spend hours alone. Sometimes, you will have to settle for minutes. You may have only a car ride as "your alone time." You have to take all the minutes you can for yourself. If you pray or believe in

a higher power, it is a great time to seek that inspirational aspect.

2. Read poems, or listen to soothing music. For some people, it is jazz, for others, it is classical music. For someone else, it may be gospel music, while for someone else, it might be gangster rap! Do what you must to prepare your mind for the journey ahead.

3. Again, research, and go back and read your notebooks. Make sure that you are prepared for all the "what if's." One of the best things you can do is to be the least surprised by an aspect of care as you can.

4. Last, be sure to chronicle the treatment in your journal. The doctors are taking notes, and so should you. You should know how your child responds to each aspect of the care so that you know how to help him or her.

These things will not ease the pain of the situation, but they will certainly help you prepare for it.

Day 10

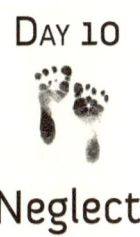

Neglect

NOTHING WAS MORE CHALLENGING for us than trying to take care of this little guy, our other children, and ourselves - talk about multi-tasking! It was inevitable for someone to get left out, and it couldn't be any of the little people. This was difficult for us because my wife and I grew up in traditional homes, where our parents often neglected themselves for us. They demonstrated an amazing level of sacrifice for both of us, and as a result, we wanted to provide the same support, and even more, for our own children. We ensured that all children had what they needed, and always asked about each other. We didn't really take ourselves into consideration.

To even think that we would be concerned with ourselves made us feel guilty and selfish. This kind of thinking was possibly one of the worst mistakes that we had made throughout our son's sickness. Many days, you could feel the tiredness, stress, and even see the physical results of our not eating, sleeping and getting proper rest. I remember looking in the mirror thinking, "Geesh, I have lost so much weight." My eyes were dark, and I looked as if I hadn't been to the barbershop for weeks. I had come to the place where all I did was go to work and the hospital. There was not time for a break, or time to consider me. I am sharing this experience with you because I do not want you to do what we did, because it was extremely unhealthy. There's not much you can do if you are not well enough to help. Also, your decisions will be affected by your self-neglect.

Not eating properly is one of the most dangerous mistakes you can make. It is imperative that you are getting as much nourishment as you can. You cannot afford to miss meals and forsake your own nutrition. Watch that self-inflicted guilt trip. I remember our son's losing his appetite - one of the side effects from the treatment. Talk about challenging! We felt so guilty every time we wanted to eat and he wasn't hungry, or even would refuse food. It just didn't seem right to eat in front of our son who couldn't eat. This was always the case. When he had an appetite (and just wasn't allowed to eat), we would just wait until we got home to eat.

The problem this presented for us is that many times, by the time we arrived at home, we were too tired to eat. I worked nights so that I could spend my days at the hospital. My wife and the staff cared for him at night. I would try to grab something light. I did not eat heavy because I didn't want to get too full and fall asleep when our son needed me to be awake. Now I am sure that sounds practical and makes complete sense to you as a parent, but it is not wise. We ran on fumes most days. We actually did not think it was at all necessary to be concerned about ourselves. As a result, we were not at our best strength, and our health suffered. We began to eat the quickest thing available to us. Unfortunately, we allowed fast food to become our friend (figuratively speaking).

One of the best things you can do for your child is to take care of yourself. We have talked about this negligence on previous days regarding other items, such as rest. Yet this nutrition policy is one that you must adopt right away.

My mom noticed that we were both declining along with our son's health - physically, emotionally, and mentally. Therefore, she decided to buy our entire family day passes to a local amusement park while she stayed with our son. She said that we needed a break and needed to take the other children, too. Mom realized that we would not have done that on our own. It didn't seem right for us to feel ok when our son didn't. It felt weird to laugh and not share it with the little guy. Mom assured us that this time would be necessary for the days ahead. That was the beginning of the pathway out of neglect for us. As a result of that one outing, my extended family and close friends decided to assist us with at least a bi-weekly "day away" from the hospital. They were even kind enough to come to the house and stay with the other children while we simply went for a walk, or went to "walk the mall." The self-neglect was finally coming to a slow stop.

I know it's hard for you to digest this right now, because every possible emotion is tugging at your heart at present. Tears fill my eyes as I write this to you, but my friend, please stop the neglect. Your child deserves all of you!

Here are some tips:

1. Keep bottled water in your car. You need to stay hydrated. Soda, coffee, and tea are not on bad for you, but they often prevent you

from getting the recommended/necessary amount of water that is needed daily.

2. Keep healthful snacks nearby. If you were already struggling with your diet, this situation could cause serious health issues for you. Use this as an opportunity to adopt some good eating habits. Travel with fruit, veggie snacks, granola bars, and even protein shakes (meal replacement drinks). These things can make a big difference in maintaining proper nutrition until you can get to a healthful meal.

3. Prepare several meals at once. I know that some people are not fans of leftovers, but in this season, they could become the family's new best friend! If you, your spouse, or a family friend can produce multiple meals at once and make the meals easy to warm up, that could be very beneficial for you and your family.

4. Don't skip breakfast! You can boil eggs while you are getting dressed in the morning. You can bake bacon (preferably turkey bacon) in

the oven while you are ironing your clothes. You can eat oatmeal with fruit. Whatever you do, make breakfast a non-negotiable part of your day.

5. Pack your lunch. Invest in a lunch box with warmers/coolers…whatever you need, but make sure you do it. There are even lunch boxes that come with slots for multiple food containers. You can pack a breakfast, lunch and dinner in it for days and nights that you will be at the hospital. You can find them in nutrition stores. Physical trainers recommend them to clients to help them get in the recommended meal count. It is recommended that you eat every 2-3 hours. You may not be able to do that, but with meal prep and planning, you can get close to achieving this recommendation. Remember that your child cannot afford risking anything to happen to you. For this reason, it is absolutely necessary that you make sure you do not neglect yourself during this crucial time.

Baby Steps

CONCLUSION

This book is an important step in a journey that my wife and I have started to encourage and educate families dealing with terminal long-term illness. We have recently launched an organization called Hinton Cares Foundation to continue helping others.

You can get additional information about the organization, future events and booking information at both:

http://tyrusjhinton.com

http://hintoncaresorganization.org

Thank you so much for your continued support.

Baby Steps

www.ingramcontent.com/pod-product-compliance
Lightning Source LLC
Chambersburg PA
CBHW020622300426
44113CB00007B/741